The Patient's Guide
CT Scan

Adam E. M. Eltorai, MD, PhD
Matthew Czar Taon, MD
Terrance T. Healey, MD

Praeclarus Press, LLC
©2019 Matthew Czar Taon. All rights reserved.

www.PraeclarusPress.com

Praeclarus Press, LLC

2504 Sweetgum Lane

Amarillo, Texas 79124 USA

806-367-9950

www.PraeclarusPress.com

DISCLAIMER
The information contained in this publication is advisory only and is not intended to replace sound clinical judgment or individualized patient care. The author disclaims all warranties, whether expressed or implied, including any warranty as the quality, accuracy, safety, or suitability of this information for any particular purpose.

ISBN: 978-1-946665-26-3

©2019 Matthew Czar Taon. All rights reserved.

Email: matthew.taon@gmail.com

Cover Design: Ken Tackett

Developmental Editing: Kathleen Kendall-Tackett

Copy Editing: Chris Tackett

Layout & Design: Nelly Murariu

CONTENTS

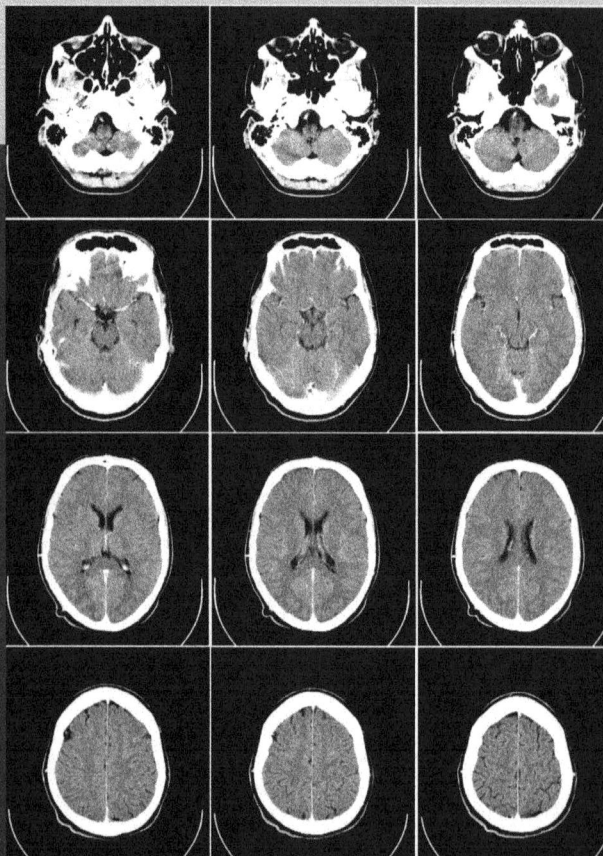

WHAT IS A "CT SCAN?"

A computerized tomography (CT) scan or (CAT) scan is a procedure in which a series of X-ray images are obtained and combined to create cross-sectional images, or slices, of your body. This allows physicians to see your internal organs to look for signs of disease. Occasionally, a contrast material (an X-ray dye) is given orally or through your veins to better visualize structures within the body. A CT scan is a quick and painless procedure that can be a very effective diagnostic tool.

The CT scanner is an open ring-like structure that resembles a giant bagel or doughnut, rather than a tunnel. Inside of this ring-like structure are devices that project and detect X-rays. As X-rays pass through the body, they are modified, and the CT scanner's X-ray detectors can measure these changes. The information collected from the X-ray detectors is transmitted to a computer that can translate the raw data into images. These images can then be examined by a radiologist (a doctor who specializes in reading medical imaging) who will be able to diagnose any possible problems.

The CT scanner uses a motorized, sliding table to move patients in and out of the machine. You may be asked to wear a gown, and remove jewelry and other metallic items to ensure image clarity. You will be asked to lie down on the exam table, remain still, and

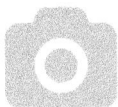

In some situations, CT scans can be used to guide minimally invasive procedures, such as biopsies, by intermittently taking pictures to assess key portions of the procedure.

possibly hold your breath for a short period of time. The scanner will often be able to acquire its images in a few seconds, although exam times vary.

Once your CT scan is complete, the images will be uploaded to the diagnostic imaging computer system for review by a diagnostic radiologist. He or she will look at the images and send a report to your healthcare provider who asked for the CT scan. Your provider will either call you or have you come in to be seen to discuss the results, typically within a week.

In some situations, CT scans can be used to guide minimally invasive procedures, such as biopsies, by intermittently taking pictures to assess key portions of the procedure. In addition, imaging from CT scans can be combined with ultrasound imaging to produce CT-ultrasound fusion imaging for procedural guidance. If you are getting a CT-guided procedure, additional information about that specific procedure will be provided.

WHY IS A CT SCAN PERFORMED?

A CT scan may be ordered by your provider for many different reasons. They are often used to evaluate the internal structures of the brain, neck, chest, abdomen, pelvis, arms, or legs. When oral contrast is administered, additional information can be obtained about the esophagus, stomach, small intestine, or large intestine. When contrast is administered through the veins, additional information can be obtained about blood vessels, lymph nodes, or vascular characteristics of soft tissues and organs.

Below is a list of common reasons to get a CT scan, though certainly not all possible reasons or conditions are covered:

- Head CT scan: To examine the brain tissue, facial bones, or skull.

- Neck CT scan: To examine the thyroid gland, lymph nodes, and neck blood vessels.

- Chest CT scan: To examine the lungs, heart, lymph nodes, and blood vessels within the chest.

- Abdominal CT scan: To examine the kidneys, liver, gallbladder, portions of the pancreas, and abdominal blood vessels.

- Pelvic CT scan: To examine the uterus, ovaries, and pelvic blood vessels.

- Upper Extremity CT scan: To examine muscles, tendons, ligaments, and blood vessels of the arms.

- Lower extremity CT scan:
  To examine muscles, tendons,
  ligaments, and blood vessels
  of the legs.

- Spine CT scan: To exam the
  bony structures of the spine.

- Dedicated vascular CT
  Angiogram: To better evaluate
  the arteries and/or veins in any
  part of the body.

Sometimes these CT scans are
looking to answer a specific
question, such as "are there
inflammatory changes around
an organ?" or "is there a mass
present?" Other times, they are
ordered to look more generally for
a problem in part of the body.

Based on the information and
concerns of the ordering provider,
the scans will be adjusted and
targeted to answer the questions
specific to your signs or symptoms.

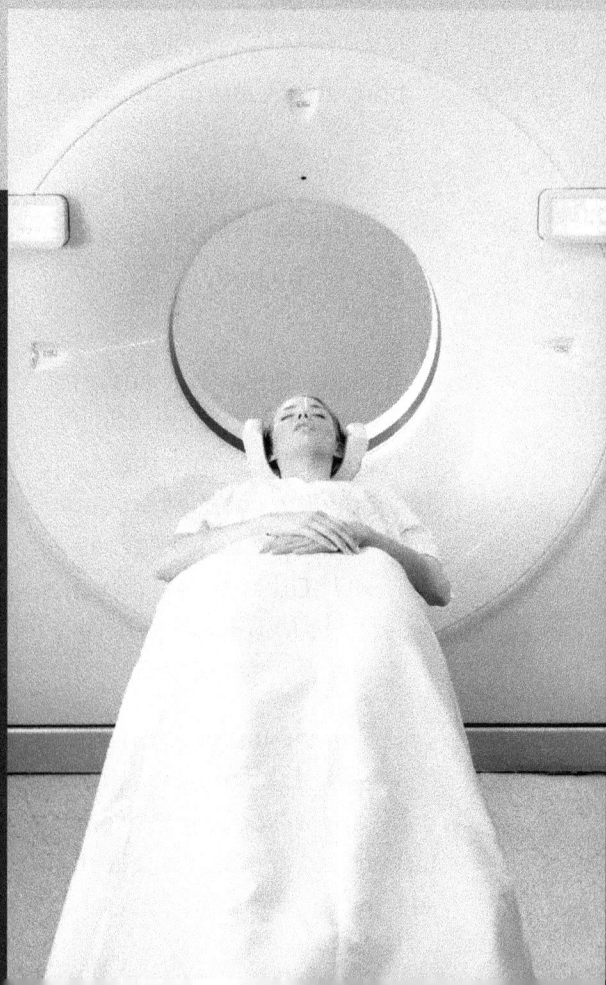

HOW DO I PREPARE FOR MY CT SCAN?

The specific preparation for a CT scan will vary based on what body part will be scanned and what questions are trying to be answered. Below, general guidelines for preparing for a CT scan are given by body part. For many CT scans, you will need to do little to no advanced preparation before the exam. Any specific preparation for your scan should be provided to you ahead of time. In most cases, you will be asked to change into a hospital gown. This ensures clarity of the CT images.

CT Head, CT Sinus, CT spine, CT Upper/ Lower Extremity without IV contrast	No preparation needed.
CT Chest *without* IV contrast	Please do not eat anything for approximately 2 hours prior to the exam. You may sip clear liquids.
CT Abdomen/ Pelvis/Kidneys/ Urinary *without* IV contrast	Please do not eat anything for approximately 4 hours prior to the exam. You may sip clear liquids.
Any CT scan *with* IV contrast	Please do not eat anything for approximately 3 hours prior to the exam. You may drink clear liquids prior to the exam. Continue to take your regular medications.

If you have a history of diabetes, high blood pressure, kidney disease, or are above 60 years of age, you may be asked to perform a creatinine blood lab test to measure your kidney function within 6 weeks prior to your CT scan.

If you have kidney failure, are on dialysis, or are on a fluid-restricted diet, please coordinate to have dialysis performed within 24 hours of your CT scan.

If you have a known allergy to IV iodinated contrast dye, it is important to communicate this to your physician or CT technologist, so you can take a corticosteroid regimen before your CT scan to prevent a contrast reaction.

If you have diabetes, it is important to stop any medication that contains Metformin at least 4 hours prior to your CT scan. Do not continue this medication until 48 hours after your CT scan. If you are taking insulin, you may continue administering this medication and may eat small snacks as necessary for insulin control.

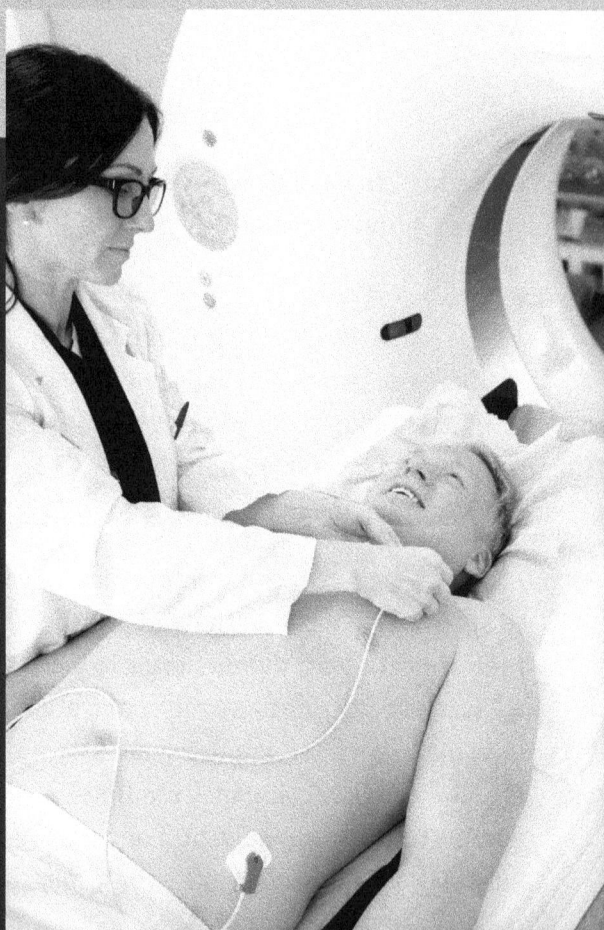

WHAT IS
THE EQUIPMENT
LIKE?

A CT scanner machine is composed of 2 main components that you will interact with: the ring-like scanner and the exam table. The ring-like structure of the CT scanner contains devices that project and detect X-rays. The information collected from the X-ray detectors is transmitted to a computer that can translate the raw data into images. The CT scanner uses a motorized, sliding table to move patients in and out of the machine. Often, this sliding table has a thick pad overlying it to provide patient comfort. A variety of pillows or foam tools may be used to optimize your positioning for the scan.

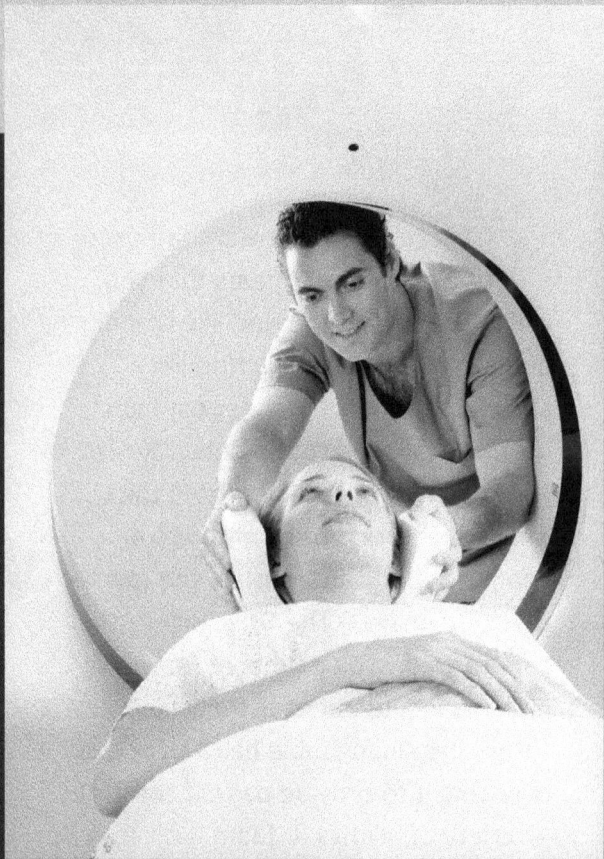

WHAT DOES THE PROCEDURE INVOLVE?

CT scans are safe and noninvasive. You will be asked to change into a hospital gown before the exam begins. You may be taken to a waiting area prior to your CT scan.

If you would like a family member or friend to accompany you and wait for you in the waiting area as you undergo your scan, you can do so for most studies.

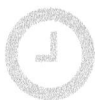

Each type of scan takes a different amount of time but usually last no more than 15 minutes.

Most scans are performed with you lying on your back on the CT exam table. Usually, the CT exam table will be moving as you are undergoing your CT scan.

Each type of scan takes a different amount of time but usually last no more than 15 minutes. The CT technologist will guide you through any movements or actions they may need you to perform, such as briefly holding your breath. The better you can follow his or her instructions, the better the quality of imaging can be obtained.

During the scan, you may be injected with contrast through your veins. As this contrast is going into your body, you may feel a warm sensation or experience a metallic taste.

WHAT DOES A CT SCAN FEEL LIKE?

CT scans are noninvasive exams and are generally painless. The only sensation that may be unpleasant involves obtaining intravenous vascular access if you need an injection of X-ray dye for an IV contrast-enhanced study.

Also, some patients may experience a warm sensation throughout the body or metallic taste once intravenous contrast is administered. This usually lasts for no more than 30 seconds.

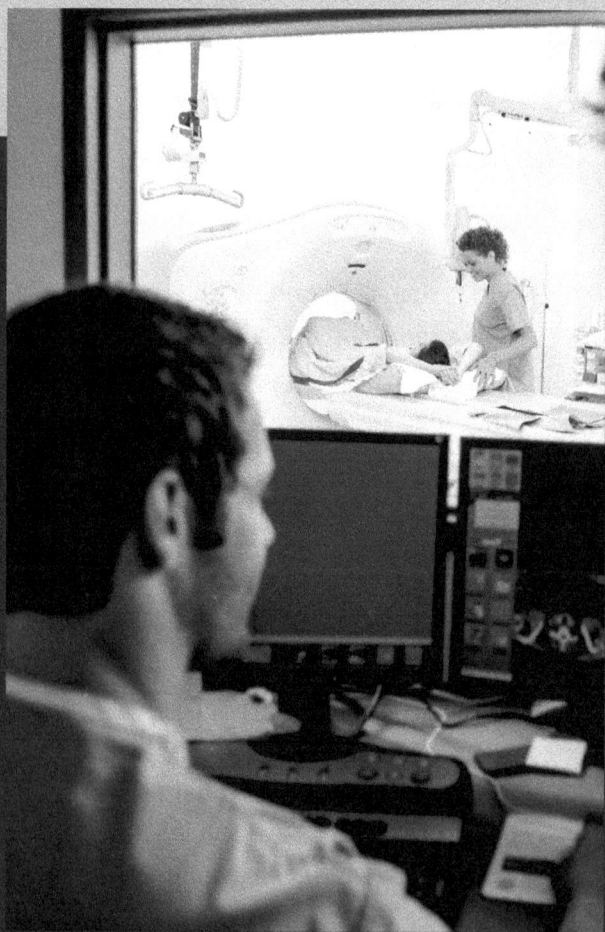

WHAT HAPPENS AFTER THE PROCEDURE?

After the CT scan procedure is complete, you will be allowed to go home and carry about your day as usual, in most cases. You are able to drive home and resume your usual diet. If you had an injection of contrast, you may be advised to slightly increase your fluid intake for the rest of the day. If you had an IV line placed, you may remove the gauze dressing from your arm after approximately 1 hour.

There are no restrictions or special instructions after someone has a CT scan, unless there was something seen that would need immediate attention or specific care. If that were the case, a practitioner will immediately let you know and speak to the doctor or provider who referred you for the scan.

If you have questions during or after the scan, you may be able to have them answered right then and there. Let your CT technician know your concerns and a provider may be able to discuss them with you during or after the CT scan.

HOW WILL I KNOW THE RESULTS OF MY CT SCAN?

Once your CT scan is finished, the images will be uploaded to the diagnostic imaging computer system for review by a diagnostic radiologist. He or she will look at the images and send a report to your healthcare provider who asked for the CT scan. Your provider will either call you or have you come in to be seen to discuss the results, typically within a week. In some cases, a radiologist can give you the results of the test right then. Other times, they need to review the case and discuss it with your doctor before the results will be available. If your results are not immediately available, it does not mean that something concerning was found; rather, it may be that the radiologist and your provider want to come up with a plan to find an explanation for your symptoms because the study was normal.

If you have questions or concerns, please let your CT technologist know, and someone should be available to talk to you.

WHAT ARE THE RISKS AND BENEFITS OF A CT SCAN?

Since CT scans use X-rays to obtain imaging, there is exposure to radiation. However, the amount of radiation is kept to a minimum by radiation dose controls on the CT scanner. Also, radiologists and CT technologists are trained in the **ALARA** principles, which recommend keeping radiation doses "As Low As Reasonably Achievable." X-rays dosage varies with each type of scan. Any small risk of cancer occurring many years or decades later is outweighed by the benefit of having an accurate diagnosis for timely treatment.

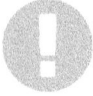

Very rarely, the iodine-based X-ray dye may cause kidney damage. The risk of this increases in patients who already have underlying kidney problems.

A contrast-enhanced CT scan uses an iodine-based intravenous X-ray dye to better visualize structures in the body. However, few people can have allergies to the iodine used in the X-ray dye. Contrast reactions may include rashes or difficulty breathing due to airway swelling. If you have had an allergic reaction to iodine or contrast dye in the past, it is extremely important to communicate this to your physician or CT technologist. In patients with prior iodine contrast allergies, a corticosteroid regimen may be administered prior to a CT scan requiring intravenous contrast, to prevent a contrast reaction.

Very rarely, the iodine-based X-ray dye may cause kidney damage. The risk of this increases in patients who already have underlying kidney problems. The risk of kidney damage due to iodine-based contrast can be decreased with adequate oral or IV hydration. Thus, patients may be asked to increase their fluid intake before and after a CT scan requiring IV contrast.

Lastly, in patients requiring an IV contrast injection, there is a risk of contrast leaking outside of the vein and into the surrounding soft tissue. This can cause temporary swelling and discomfort, which can often be treated with warm compresses.

Are there limitations to a CT scan?

CT scans are very effective for evaluating many different medical conditions, but they are not perfect. The primary limitations relate to patient motion artifact, metallic density artifact, lack of intravenous contrast, and signal-to-noise ratio. These will affect what can be seen, how well things can be seen, and how clearly the images can be interpreted.

When patients are moving during a CT scan, this will produce motion artifact and blur the subsequent CT images. The motion of the diaphragm during breathing can also produce motion artifact. This is the reason why some studies, namely CT scans of the chest and abdomen, require patients to briefly hold their breath, to limit motion artifact. Other studies, such as CT head and spine, are not really affected by respiratory motion but can be severely limited if the patient is moving the rest of their body.

Metallic hardware or foreign objects within the body can disrupt the imaging of a CT scan and limit proper evaluation of adjacent tissues.

Some disease processes require intravenous contrast for proper evaluation. However, if

Metallic hardware or foreign objects within the body can disrupt the imaging of a CT scan and limit proper evaluation of adjacent tissues.

intravenous contrast was not administered for whatever reason, evaluation can be severely limited.

All imaging, whether it involves X-rays, ultrasound, or MRI, utilizes a concept of signal-to-noise ratio to differentiate between useful imaging data (signal) and useless information (noise). In CT scans where there is a high signal-to-noise ratio, there is a clear distinction between important structures. In CT scans where there is a low signal-to-noise ratio, there may be blurring of important structures with non-important structures. The signal-to-noise ratio can be affected by many technical aspects of the exam, including how much radiation exposure is utilized and the patient's body habitus. In studies with a low signal-to-noise ratio, effective evaluation of the imaging can be severely limited.

FREQUENTLY ASKED QUESTIONS

Does a CT scan involve any radiation?

Yes. CT scans use X-rays to obtain images, which exposes you to radiation. Radiologists and radiation technologists are trained to be cognizant of the ALARA principles, which encourage radiation dosages to be "as low as reasonably achievable."

Are there any risks to a CT scan?

Yes. Risks include radiation exposure, which has a low risk of causing cancer many years to decades later, iodine contrast allergy, contrast-induced renal injury, and contrast-leaking from the IV access site.

How long will my CT scan take?

It varies based on the study but usually less than 15 minutes for an exam.

When will my results be available?

It varies based on the study, but you should have results within a week.

Can I obtain a CT scan if I am pregnant?

According to the American College of Radiology, no single diagnostic X-ray has a radiation dose significant enough to cause adverse effects in a developing embryo or fetus. In general, however, CT scans are not recommended during pregnancy unless the benefits of the CAT scan clearly outweigh the potential risk.

GLOSSARY

ALARA

"As low as reasonably achievable."

ARTIFACT

Any part of an image that does not accurately represent the anatomic structures present within the subject being.

BIOPSY

An examination of tissue removed from a living body to discover the presence, cause, or extent of a disease.

CROSS-SECTIONAL IMAGING

A term usually used to refer to CT, MRI, ultrasound, and related imaging techniques that view the body in slices.

INTRAVENOUS

A term meaning "through or within the veins."

TOMOGRAPHY

A phrase meaning imaging by sections. The Greek word *tomos* means slice/section.

VASCULAR/VASCULATURE

A term indicating involvement of the arteries or veins.

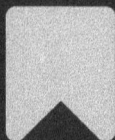

ADDITIONAL RESOURCES

Radiologyinfo.org

http://www.jacr.org/content/acr-patient-summaries?underjournal

American College of Radiology Patient and Family Resources

https://www.acr.org/Practice-Management-Quality-Informatics/Practice-Toolkit/Patient-Resources

Topics in Radiology Safety

https://www.radiologyinfo.org/en/submenu.cfm?pg=safety

MY CONTACTS

NAME

CONTACT

NAME

CONTACT

NAME

CONTACT

NAME

CONTACT

MY APPOINTMENTS

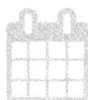

MONDAY
Date:
_____

THURSDAY
Date:
_____

TUESDAY
Date:
_____

FRIDAY
Date:
_____

WEDNESDAY
Date:
_____

SATURDAY
Date:
_____

MY QUESTIONS

MY QUESTIONS

MY NOTES

MY NOTES

MY NOTES

MY NOTES

MY NOTES

MY NOTES